UNDERSTANDING YOUR
DIABETES

FOR PEOPLE WITH
NON-INSULIN-
DEPENDENT
(TYPE 2) DIABETES

Acknowledgements

The author acknowledges with appreciation the constructive criticism of the many patients, nurses and other health professionals who helped to produce this book. Special thanks go to Eleanor Baldwin who provided nutritional information for this book.

UNDERSTANDING YOUR
DIABETES

DR PH WISE

MB, PhD, FRCP, FRACP
CONSULTANT PHYSICIAN IN ENDOCRINOLOGY

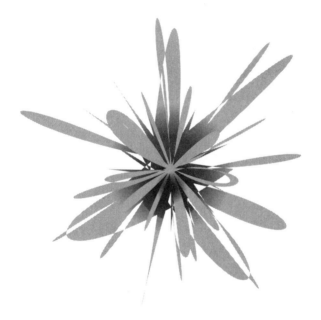

FOR PEOPLE WITH
NON-INSULIN-
DEPENDENT
(TYPE 2) DIABETES

foulsham
LONDON • NEW YORK • TORONTO • SYDNEY

foulsham

The Publishing House, Bennetts Close,
Cippenham, Berkshire SL1 5AP, England

ISBN 0-572-02547-5

Printed in Great Britain by St. Edmundsbury Press, Bury St. Edmunds, Suffolk.

Introduction

You may have had diabetes for some time; perhaps you already know much of what is in this book. On the other hand, the diagnosis may have just been made, and all that is involved in coming to terms with your condition may seem a little bewildering.

This book has been written to give you some idea of what diabetes is all about. It tries to answer the type of questions you will ask, both now and in the future, in order to help you understand and cope with non-insulin-dependent (type 2) diabetes. It cannot cover the whole subject and makes no attempt to replace the advice and guidance of your physician. You will also find a list of further reading at the back of this book.

There is one thing that most authorities agree upon: the more that people with diabetes know and understand about their disorder, the better they will be able to control their illness and the healthier they are likely to be. Hopefully, this book will go some way towards achieving that, but never hesitate to ask for additional information and help whenever you feel you need it.

1

What is diabetes?

Diabetes is the name given to a disturbed chemical balance in the body, which can affect a number of different organs. The word diabetes comes from a Greek expression meaning 'siphon'. It refers to the increased urination and thirst which often occurs in newly diagnosed or uncontrolled cases. These symptoms are due to the high glucose content in the urine. The sugar in the urine drags water out with it, the body gets dry and you feel thirsty. All this follows an excessive build-up of glucose in the blood, because there is not enough insulin in your body to deal with it. Diabetes is due to partial or complete lack of insulin. This hormone is normally released directly into the blood circulation from small pockets of cells called Islets of Langerhans, which are scattered throughout the pancreas gland (sweetbread). The pancreas rests in the upper abdomen, just beneath the liver, partly behind the stomach in the loop of the duodenum (see diagram opposite).

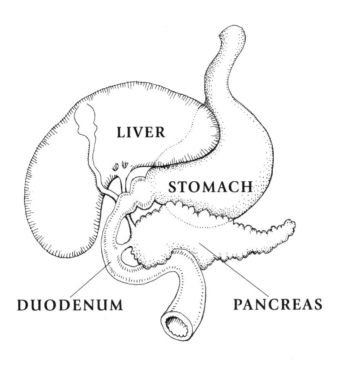

LIVER

STOMACH

DUODENUM   PANCREAS

The pancreas also produces enzymes, which pass through a duct into the duodenum, where they assist with the digestion of food. This part of the pancreas is only rarely affected in diabetes. Insulin in usable form was first extracted from animal pancreas in 1921 by two Canadians, Banting and Best. Shortly afterwards it proved successful in the treatment of human diabetes. About one person in every 50 is diabetic. Most can be treated without the need for insulin injections.

2

How is food normally processed?

All foods contain one or more energy-producing substances called carbohydrates, proteins and fats. Once absorbed through the small intestine, they are all processed in the liver, where all three can be converted to glucose, and then released into the bloodstream. However, carbohydrates, especially in a refined form such as sugar and sweets, are the most rapidly absorbed. Accordingly, they produce the biggest rises in blood glucose level. Any rise in blood glucose 'triggers' the islets of the pancreas to produce insulin, which is then released into the blood vessels passing through the pancreas. In this way, insulin can find its way through the blood circulation to all other body tissues.

Although insulin has many different effects, it has one main action: to help glucose in the blood to enter the tissue cells, where it is used as a source of energy. If not required for immediate energy production, insulin also ensures that glucose is converted either to glycogen (for short term energy storage), or to fat (for more long term energy storage).

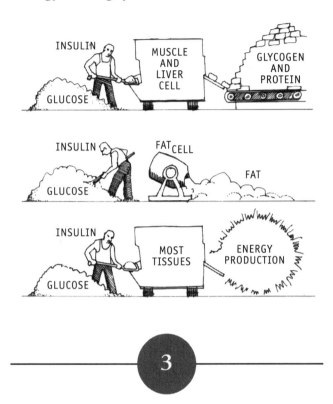

3

Why does diabetes develop?

Diabetes is partly inherited, even though you may not be aware that your ancestors were affected. Where diabetes begins before the age of 40, lack of insulin is often complete, perhaps resulting from additional severe damage to the pancreas gland by a virus. Symptoms are then commonly sudden and severe, and for these people with so-called type 1 diabetes, only insulin itself can be used for treatment.

However, in the case of maturity onset, non-insulin-dependent or type 2 diabetes, insulin deficiency is often only mild. Of equal importance is the fact that insulin is being prevented from acting properly on the body's cells. This so-called insulin resistance may be purely inherited, but can also develop because you have become overweight, or because of the effects of ageing or certain drugs. It may also have resulted from some form of stress such as anxiety, infection or some other illness.

In all of these situations, the body's need for insulin is increased, but cannot be satisfied by the faulty islets. The end result is that glucose in the blood cannot properly enter tissue cells. Therefore its level in the blood remains above normal, even when you have not had anything to eat. After food, blood glucose levels rise even higher and remain raised for longer. Such rises of blood sugar above normal are referred to as hyperglycaemia.

What symptoms does uncontrolled diabetes (hyperglycaemia) produce?

In the early stages, or if the build-up of glucose is only slight, there may be **no symptoms at all.** As the glucose level rises higher, one or more of the following may occur:

❖ The lens of the eye may alter its shape, producing **blurring** of vision.

❖ High glucose levels in the blood reduce the body's defences against **infection**, particularly in the skin, urine and lungs. In fact, it may have been a severe or chronic infection which first alerted your doctor that you might have diabetes.

❖ By overflowing into the urine (where it can be easily tested), glucose may draw water with it: **more urine** is then passed.

❖ Passing more urine draws on the body's fluid reserves and causes **thirst** in an attempt by the body to replace lost fluid.

❖ Excessive urination also results in loss of essential chemicals (sodium, potassium and magnesium), producing **cramps, tiredness and weakness, and weight loss.**

❖ If severe loss of fluid occurs in the urine, the body becomes dry **(dehydration);** breathlessness and even coma may then occur. Fortunately this is uncommon in your type of diabetes.

What is a normal blood glucose level?

In people without diabetes, the fasting blood glucose level (after not eating overnight) is less than 5 millimoles per litre, or 90 milligrams per decilitre (shortened to mmol/l or mg/dl). After food, it rarely rises above 8mmol/l (145mg/dl). In untreated or uncontrolled diabetes it can rise to 30mmol/l (540mg/dl) or even higher. Your doctor will probably aim to keep your blood glucose level below 10mmol/l (180mg/dl) for most of the time and in some cases will help you to achieve the lower (more normal) levels mentioned above. It is important to realise that the symptoms of diabetes (see page 11) are unlikely to

Normal variation of blood glucose in a non-diabetic person

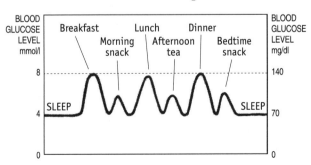

occur unless your blood glucose is consistently higher than 14mmol/l (250mg/dl).

You may feel well, but this does not necessarily indicate that your diabetes is controlled.

6

Does diabetes ever go away?

No. It can always be controlled and with treatment you should feel completely well. Even when treated, however, you must still carefully watch your condition and ensure that it is regularly reviewed by your doctor for the rest of your life.

7

What are the major aims and principles of diabetic treatment?

The first aim of treating your diabetes is to keep your blood glucose level as close as possible to that of a non-diabetic person. By this and other means, the second aim can be achieved: to minimise or avoid the so-called complications of diabetes (see question 23 on pages 41–6).

Treatment of your type of diabetes is quite simple – particularly when over-weight is a factor. Such an increase in weight is due mainly to a combination of eating more food than the body needs, together with insufficient exercise, although some people certainly do seem to gain weight more easily than others, especially as they get older. You have an excellent chance of treating your diabetes by eating less food, possibly of better quality, and by exercising more. Your doctor will arrange for you to see a dietitian for advice on the food that you should include in your daily diet. Sometimes it is necessary to prescribe additional tablets to achieve full control of your diabetes. This will be discussed later (see question 12 on pages 25–8).

8

What are the principles of diabetic diets?

A diabetic diet is a healthy, balanced diet; the sort of diet that is recommended for everyone (although very young children and babies have special requirements). Why not convert your family and friends? Your dietitian, ideally also involving some members of your family, will tell you about foods which will suit both your likes and needs, whatever your ethnic or national background. There is no need to buy 'special' diabetic foods; they are more expensive, and not necessarily more healthy.

Some foods cause problems by causing a very large rise in blood glucose. They are then said to have a high glycaemic index (GI). In general, there are alternatives that are healthier, not only for people with diabetes but for good nutrition generally. Your dietitian will explain this to you in more detail, and will be able to provide you with a list that will help you to choose foods of low glycaemic index. There are six general principles that all people with diabetes should follow to keep their diabetes well controlled.

Reduce sugar and sugary foods.
We are talking mainly about glucose itself, jam, honey, sweets, chocolates, fizzy (sugary) drinks, and fruit squashes or juices. These foods cause a rapid rise in blood glucose which is difficult for insulin to deal with. Many foods contain sugar (chemical name: sucrose). We now know that sucrose has quite a low glycaemic index and only makes your blood glucose go half as high as glucose itself. However, sucrose gives you 'empty calories' – they have very little nutritional value. It is therefore wise to avoid foods in which sugar is the major ingredient. Check the ingredient label of a food if you are not sure whether it is suitable. The ingredients are listed in order of weight, so if sugar is at the top of the list, it means the food contains a large amount. If sugar is towards the end of the list, the food is suitable as it contains very little sugar. Artificial sweeteners are safe, but avoid those that are combined with sugar.

Eat regularly.
You should aim for three meals a day. One or two large meals raise the blood glucose too high and are difficult for insulin to deal with properly. A meal may be as little as a sandwich, or as much as a cooked meal of meat, potatoes and vegetables, followed by dessert. Eating regularly is particularly important to avoid **hypoglycaemia** (a hypo or low blood sugar). If you are being treated with diet only, this will not happen. However, if you are taking any of the tablets in the first group of drugs mentioned later (question 12 on page 26), a hypo may occur if you do not eat regularly.

Eating a larger meal than usual is fine, on occasions, but you may need to increase your tablet dose. Your diabetes nurse, doctor, or dietitian will be able to advise you on this.

Eat some starchy food with each meal.
In earlier years, people with diabetes were advised to avoid or restrict all starches. We now know that a certain intake of starches is important. They are broken down into sugar by the body. The healthier types are broken down more slowly than sugary foods, causing a slower, smaller rise in blood

glucose. Some starches should be included in each meal. Boiled potatoes, oatmeal or multigrain breads, oat-based cereals, such as porridge, All Bran and muesli, and brown rice are the ones to go for. A low blood glucose level or hypo (see question 13 on page 28) may occur if you forget to include these foods or try to reduce them drastically.

However, you should note that white bread and baked potatoes have a very high glycaemic index; avoid them! These foods, together with white rice and some refined cereals like cornflakes, are likely to contribute to poor diabetic control. They may well cause weight gain as well.

Eat less fat and fatty foods.

We are including here butter, oil, margarine, all fried foods and pastry of all types. Having a high fat intake increases your risk of suffering from heart attacks or strokes, which are in any case rather more likely to occur in someone with diabetes. Smoking or being overweight increases the risk still further. It makes sense to cut down risks! Reducing fat has the added advantage that it automatically reduces your calorie intake. Weight for weight, high-fat foods may have as many as twice the number of calories than non-fat or low-fat alternatives. Avoiding high-fat foods will therefore help you to reduce your weight, if necessary, or help to prevent you from becoming overweight.

Drink alcohol in moderation.
There is no uniform agreement on safe alcohol limits: however, safe weekly limits are generally considered to be 15–18 units for a woman, or 22–28 units for a man, spread over the week. One unit is a single pub measure of spirit, an average glass of wine or a half pint of beer, lager or cider. Alcohol is high in calories and will make you gain weight. Too much of it is also bad for your liver, heart, brain and nerves. The actual amount of alcohol that will cause damage to different people will vary considerably, however.

Alcohol excess is particularly harmful if nerve damage from diabetes is already present (see page 43). Too much alcohol at once, especially on an empty stomach, may actually cause your blood glucose level to go too low. **Do not drink alcohol on an empty stomach,** avoid having more than three or four drinks in a session, and always follow alcohol with a snack containing at least some starchy food, such as a sandwich. This is particularly important at bedtime, to avoid having low blood glucose levels overnight.

Eat more fibre.
Dietary fibre is the part of a plant that is not digested properly by the body. High-fibre foods include multi-grain bread, brown long-grain rice (which has a lower glycaemic index than white rice), wholegrain pasta, vegetables (especially beans, peas and lentils) and wholegrain breakfast cereals. Eating high-fibre foods with your meals reduces the rise in blood sugar that occurs after eating. High-fibre foods can also be helpful in reducing blood cholesterol, and also tend to be quite filling. They can therefore be helpful in reducing weight and preventing weight gain. They also help to produce regular bowel movements.

Not being overweight has been mentioned many times in this section. Turn to page 23 to see the desirable weight for you. It is very important that you try to reduce your weight if you are overweight. Diabetes is more difficult to control when you are overweight. If you are having difficulty in losing weight, ask your doctor to refer you to the dietitian. They will draw up an eating plan tailored to your needs that will help you to achieve your weight target.

It is very important to see a dietitian regularly; you will be given a lot of information and no one would expect you to remember it all at your first visit. Furthermore, the diet may need to be changed over a period of time – particularly if you change your way of life, gain weight, or if the type of insulin you use is changed. Check page 60 to be sure you have a contact number for your dietician.

9

Is weight control important?

Yes. Being overweight increases your need for insulin and can make your diabetes less stable. It may also cause or aggravate conditions unrelated to diabetes, such as high blood pressure and arthritis. The only way you can influence your weight is by diet and exercise. Remember that one extra hour of brisk walking (or half an hour of continuous swimming, jogging or squash) each day will almost predictably allow you to lose about 7 kg (15 lb) in a year – providing you do not increase your food intake! Use the table below as a guide to your ideal weight which should ideally be towards the centre of the range for your height.

Guide to healthy weight range for adult men and women

HEIGHT		HEALTHY WEIGHT RANGE	
4' 10"	146 cm	6 st 10 lb–8 st 4 lb	43–53 kg
4' 11"	149 cm	7 st 0 lb–8 st 8 lb	44–55 kg
5' 0"	152 cm	7 st 4 lb–9 st 2 lb	46–58 kg
5' 1"	154 cm	7 st 7 lb–9 st 5 lb	47–60 kg
5' 2"	157 cm	7 st 10 lb–9 st 12 lb	49–63 kg
5' 3"	160 cm	7 st 13 lb–10 st 2 lb	50–64 kg
5' 4"	162 cm	8 st 4 lb–10 st 7 lb	52–67 kg
5' 5"	164 cm	8 st 7 lb–10 st 10 lb	53–68 kg
5' 6"	166 cm	8 st 10 lb–11 st 0 lb	55–70 kg
5' 7"	169 cm	8 st 12 lb–11 st 5 lb	56–72 kg
5' 8"	172 cm	9 st 0 lb–11 st 10 lb	58–75 kg
5' 9"	175 cm	9 st 4 lb–12 st 0 lb	59–77 kg
5' 10"	177 cm	9 st 8 lb–12 st 6 lb	61–79 kg
5' 11"	179 cm	9 st 12 lb–12 st 8 lb	64–80 kg
6' 0"	182 cm	10 st 2 lb–12 st 12 lb	65–82 kg
6' 1"	184 cm	10 st 7 lb–13 st 4 lb	67–84 kg
6' 2"	187 cm	10 st 12 lb–13 st 10 lb	69–87 kg

Figures given are for a recommended body mass index (BMI) of 20–25 calculated as weight (in kg) divided by height (in metres)^2.

Is exercise important?

Yes. Any form of exercise causes the muscles to use more glucose. In fact, lack of exercise is now thought to be one of the major reasons why diabetes is becoming more common. Not only is the blood glucose level lowered immediately after exercise, but there appears to be a long-term lowering of blood glucose in people whose lifestyle is more energetic. Most people do not realise how inactive they really are. Tiredness and fatigue after a day's work are more likely to be due to emotional stress and tension than to the effects of muscular exercise. Any type of moderate exercise is satisfactory, including cycling, regular sport, or just plain walking. A careful look at your lifestyle and discussion with friends and family should help you plan a more energetic way of life, regardless of your age or any medical problems.

What if diet and exercise alone are not sufficient?

Provided that your symptoms are not severe, your doctor and dietitian will probably persevere for several weeks just watching the effects of their advice on diet and exercise, particularly if you are very much overweight. If control is not achieved in this way (as shown by consistently high urine or blood glucose levels), or if your first symptoms are quite severe, additional tablets will be prescribed. Insulin itself cannot be taken by mouth, since it is destroyed by enzymes in the stomach and bowel.

How do 'anti-diabetic' tablets (oral hypoglycaemic drugs) work?

Anti-diabetic drugs can be divided into four distinct groups.

The first group

The first group of drugs is listed below.

Chemical name	Trade name
Tolbutamide	Rastinon
	Pramide
	Artosin
Chlorpropamide	Diabenese
Glibenclamide	Euglucon
	Daonil
Gliquidone	Glurenorm
Glipizide	Glibenese
	Minodiab
Tolazamide	Tolanase
Gliclazide	Diamicron
Glimepiride	Amaryl
Repaglinide	Novonorm

All the drugs in this group act partly by stimulating the pancreas to produce more insulin, and in some cases by improving the action of whatever insulin is already being produced. Repaglinide is included in this group since it has a similar action on the islets of the pancreas, although its chemical structure is different to the other (sulphonylurea) drugs in the group.

Some of these drugs have other effects that benefit diabetes. These are still under study. Some drugs have a very short-lasting action (tolbutamide, glimepiride and repaglinide); chlorpropamide has a particularly long-lasting action. Your doctor will choose one that is suited to your particular condition and lifestyle.

The second group
The second group of drugs are called biguanides, the only one currently in use being metformin (Glucophage). This acts by improving the action of any insulin you are still producing, directly helping glucose to enter tissue cells. It also stops the liver from producing glucose.

The third group
The third group of drugs are called alpha-glucosidase inhibitors, the current main member of which is called acarbose (Glucobay). These drugs act by slowing down the breakdown of complex carbohydrates such as starches. The glucose that results from the breakdown will then be absorbed more slowly.

The fourth group
The fourth group of drugs are called glitazones. These are not yet available in all countries. These drugs work by

helping insulin to perform its main job: getting glucose into the cells of your body. By helping to correct abnormal blood fat levels, they may also reduce the risk of heart attack and stroke.

13

Can tablets ever produce side effects?

Sulphonylureas (and **repaglinide**) when given in too high a dose can cause the blood glucose level to drop too far (hypoglycaemia or 'hypo'). Glimepiride and tolbutamide are probably the least likely to cause this problem. A hypo may produce a feeling of hunger, dizziness, slurred speech, trembling, sweating, faintness, or even loss of consciousness. The blood glucose level usually drops to below 2.5mmol/l (45mg/dl) in someone who is having a hypo. Clearly, if you miss a meal, a hypo is more likely to occur and irregular or missed meals must particularly be avoided with glibenclamide and chlorpropamide. All these drugs can occasionally produce a rash. In some people taking sulphonylureas (especially chlorpropamide), even a small alcoholic drink can produce a hot flush. If this occurs, tell your doctor; you can then be prescribed a different tablet in the same group.

Metformin only lowers the blood glucose too far if it is used in combination with other glucose-lowering drugs. However, it can produce a feeling of sickness, stomach discomfort or diarrhoea. This feeling may wear off in a couple of weeks, or can be relieved by reducing the dose. However, if abdominal symptoms persist, contact your doctor. Very rarely, it can produce serious illness, particularly if there are other heart, liver, kidney, or blood vessel problems. Your doctor will regularly check for these other problems and will not prescribe metformin if any are present.

Acarbose (Glucobay) may produce excessive wind, and sometimes diarrhoea. Other than this, it is quite safe.

Some **glitazones** may damage the liver, and therefore may not be given if there is already some evidence of liver problem. Your doctor will regularly check liver function. If drugs in this group are used with insulin or oral anti-diabetic drugs, it can increase your chance of having a hypo.

14

Can hypos do any harm?

They certainly can. You can lose concentration while doing an important task like driving a car, and even lose consciousness altogether. There is also some evidence that repeated hypos may cause permanent brain damage, particularly as you get older. More emphasis is now being placed on achieving lower blood glucose levels to prevent longer-term complications (see question 23 on page 41); therefore there is a rather greater risk of having a hypo. The occasional hypo may be unavoidable, due to a late meal. However, the early symptoms must be treated promptly, so **always** have some Dextrosol or a small carton of fruit juice in your pocket or bag. Also make sure that you have some identification on you to say that you have diabetes: a card is not as good as a pendant or bracelet (see page 57).

What happens if the tablets do not work?

You must first ask yourself if you are still keeping to the programme of diet and exercise prescribed for you. Remember that the tablets are not substitutes for this programme. If you are doing all the right things and control is still poor, your doctor may suggest an increased tablet dose or a change of tablets, perhaps adding metformin or acarbose to a sulphonylurea drug. Insulin injections may be recommended.

Commencing on insulin is not a calamity. Up to 60 per cent of people with diabetes who are initially not insulin-dependent may need insulin at some time if blood glucose control is not satisfactory. Most people will actually feel very much better once insulin is begun. Sometimes your doctor may add a dose of insulin to your existing tablet routine, either in the morning or in the evening. On the other hand, insulin may be given instead of the tablets. The routine of giving injections every day can be rapidly mastered even by the most elderly person, perhaps with the help of a district nurse or relative. Ask your doctor for the companion volume to this book, which deals with insulin-dependent (type 1) diabetes, if insulin is in fact needed.

16

How can I tell whether my diabetes is actually controlled?

By the way I feel?
No! This can be most unreliable method. Most people with diabetes can feel perfectly well even if their diabetes is not controlled; yet this state of affairs can produce undesirable effects over time. These are dealt with in question 23 on page 41. You should be able to recognise easily the symptoms listed in question 4 on page 11. If they occur, your diabetes is seriously out of control! The cause must be found and corrected immediately.

By testing for glucose in the urine?
Yes. All people with diabetes should test their own urine at the very least

once each day. Positive tests usually mean that the diabetes has not been well controlled during the previous four or five hours. Even negative tests may not give the whole picture: blood glucose can be quite high without it showing up in the urine (see question 18 on page 35).

By testing for glucose in the blood?
Yes. Measuring the blood glucose levels is the most direct way of checking how good the control of your diabetes really is. You can do blood tests yourself, as explained later (see page 37), again ideally once or twice each day. However, your doctor may not feel that self-testing of blood glucose is necessary for you; for many people with diabetes, regular urine tests are adequate. The diagram on page 13 gave you an idea how, in a person who does not have diabetes, blood glucose levels rise in response to food, and return to normal as the body's insulin takes effect. In a person with diabetes, a blood glucose level that is mostly below 10mmol/l (180mg/dl) is a good target. Your doctor or diabetes nurse will advise you on what your personal targets should be.

By testing the HbA1c?

Yes. This is a blood test that is taken by your doctor or nurse and analysed by the laboratory. The result of the test gives an estimate of how well your diabetes has been controlled over the previous two to three months. Ask your doctor what your level is, so that you know how you are getting on with your control. People without diabetes usually have levels below 6 per cent. Levels above 7 per cent usually mean that there is room for improvement! Some doctors prefer the fructosamine test. This measures diabetic control over the previous 10 to 14 days.

17

How do I test the urine?

There are two appropriate methods. Whichever test is used, it is most important that you follow the instructions exactly: although they are simple to do, you can still get a wrong answer if you don't do the test carefully!

Clinistix

These dip-strips only tell you whether or not glucose is present in the urine. They are not accurate enough to tell you the actual amount and are therefore unsatisfactory for routine use by people with diabetes.

Diabur or Diastix dip-strips

These show a clearer and more definite colour change, depending on exactly how much glucose is present in the urine. They are quite satisfactory for routine use. The result should be recorded as 0, $\frac{1}{10}$, 1 per cent, and so on.

18

What does glucose in the urine really mean?

Consider the glucose levels in the blood to be like water in a tank. When it reaches a certain level (the threshold), it overflows into the urine. In most people this threshold is above 8mmol/l (140mg/dl), shown by A in the figure on page 36. This is the highest blood glucose level reached by most non-diabetics (and people with

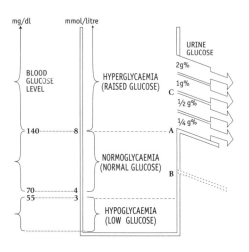

well controlled diabetes). **Therefore, absence of glucose in the urine usually means good diabetic control; the worse the control, the more glucose will appear in the urine.**

However, your threshold may be low (B in figure); then glucose may be present in the urine even with a normal blood glucose level. Finally, your threshold may be high (C in the figure). Then the blood glucose levels can be quite high without it showing up in the urine. You will therefore be misled into thinking that your diabetes is well controlled. It is partly for these reasons that your doctor may advise you to test your blood rather than your urine. It is also worth remembering that people without diabetes do not have sugar in their urine; ideally, you should be aiming for this target too!

How do I test my blood?

Pricking your finger yourself is not such an ordeal if you use one of the newer pricking devices fitted with a lancet. The technique is easily shown to you by your doctor or nurse. Place a drop of blood on the end of a special glucose testing strip and the colour change allows quite an accurate assessment of your blood glucose level. Be careful to get a good drop of blood (not a smear). For many strips, it is also essential that you wipe the blood off the strip at exactly the right time recommended by the manufacturers, otherwise an inaccurate result is obtained. Meters are available to give a digital read-out of your sugar level. They are quite inexpensive and some have built-in timing devices too, together with a memory bank, so that you do not need to write down the result immediately. Whichever test is used, it is most important that you follow the instructions very carefully.

When should urine or blood be tested?

Preferably every day. First thing in the morning (or before a meal) is the time when glucose in blood and urine is likely to be at its lowest level; one or two hours after the main meal of the day is the time when the glucose level is likely to be at its highest. Both these measurements are important, and your doctor will recommend tests spread throughout the day to get a clear picture of what is going on.

It is essential that you write the test results down in a record book and bring this either to the clinic or to your doctor's surgery each time you visit. In this way, the doctor or nurse can see how well you are controlled and can provide suggestions as to how control may be improved.

What level of control should I be aiming for?

The best possible! We have always considered that lower blood glucose levels mean less damage in the long run to the eyes, kidneys and nerves. A recent large research project called the United Kingdom Prospective Diabetes Study (UKPDS) has proved this beyond doubt. In addition, this study showed a reduced risk of heart attack with better diabetes control and less likelihood of needing an operation for cataracts. The target HbA1c (see page 34) is 7 per cent; 6 per cent is even better! However, even if this result is not readily attainable, every 0.5 per cent improvement from what you have at the moment is worthwhile and will reduce the risks of these complications. Ask your doctor to check your HbA1c regularly, so that you can monitor your progress.

If you are checking urine glucose, negative tests before and two hours after your main meal means that your diabetes is probably well controlled. If you check blood glucose levels, then before meal levels of less than 7mmol/l (125mg/dl) and levels of less than 10mmol/l (180mg/dl) two hours after meals are worth aiming for.

22

What can cause diabetes to go out of control?

There are many things that affect the blood glucose level: the tug-of-war diagram on page 41 will help remind you of the most important ones. If you keep this model in mind, it will help you to achieve the best control under all circumstances.

It is most important to remember that even a slight infection like a bad cold can affect your control quite badly. This will show up as a positive urine test or a high blood glucose level. Emotional stresses do the same thing. If your tests run high, contact your doctor or Hotline number (see page 59); you may need a bigger dose of tablets or even a short course of insulin until the problem settles down.

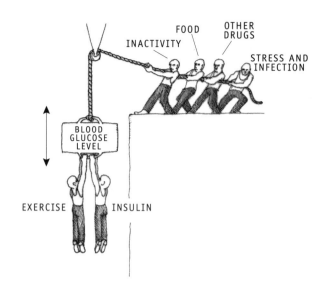

FOOD
INACTIVITY
OTHER DRUGS
STRESS AND INFECTION
BLOOD GLUCOSE LEVEL
EXERCISE   INSULIN

23

What are the so-called complications of diabetes?

Arteriosclerosis

Arteriosclerosis (hardening of the arteries) occurs to some extent in almost every person as they age, whether they are diabetic or not. In people with diabetes, it tends to occur somewhat earlier than usual. Arteriosclerosis is the cause of strokes and heart attacks. It may also produce poor circulation in the legs, which leads to painful calves on walking, poor healing of abrasions and blisters, and occasionally gangrene. Hardening of the arteries is caused by fat being deposited in the walls of the arteries so that they become narrowed and even blocked. From time to time, your doctor will check the level of cholesterol (as well as other fats) in your blood. Keeping these blood fat levels normal is now known to reduce the risk of developing heart attacks and strokes. The way to keep the fat levels normal is to keep to your recommended diet (see question 8 on page 15). Somewhat stricter dieting and even medicines may be prescribed for you if the fats in the blood test are found to be above safe levels. **People with diabetes should not smoke.** Smoking is the other big cause of hardening of the arteries. If arteries do become blocked, they can quite often be treated by a surgeon stretching or bypassing the block. But prevention is better than cure!

Cataracts

Cataracts are degenerative changes in the lens of the eye which can cause dimness of vision. Cataracts occur commonly in all people and somewhat more frequently in people with diabetes, especially if blood sugar levels are allowed to run high. Cataracts can be treated by quite a simple operation: the surgeon will usually replace your damaged lens with an artificial one.

Retinopathy

Retinopathy is the name given to leaky and abnormally fragile small blood vessels in the retina, the seeing part of the eye. In some people with diabetes such abnormalities may cause blurring, and occasionally loss of vision. In the early stages, however, you may not be aware that the retina is being damaged. It is therefore up to you to make sure that a doctor (or suitably qualified optician) checks your eyes every year with an ophthalmoscope. Drops will often be put in the eyes to widen the pupils and provide a better view of your retinas. Even once retinopathy has developed, it can be treated by using laser beam therapy – unless it is left too late. Again, think of prevention. Lower blood or urine glucose levels and a lower blood pressure (see question 24 on page 46) mean a much lower risk of retinal damage.

Neuropathy

Neuropathy signifies nerve damage, which can cause weakness, pins and needles or a loss of feeling in the feet or hands. Some people have leg pains or feel that they are walking on cotton wool. You may not be aware that you have a loss of feeling in the feet; only a regular check by your doctor will make it possible to pick this problem up in its earliest form. Occasionally, dizziness and other unusual symptoms may occur. Even impotence can develop, although this may be due to factors other than diabetes. If you have this problem, do discuss it with you doctor, since many possible treatments for this are now available.

Nephropathy

Nephropathy means kidney damage, and may occur after long-standing diabetes. It is for this reason that your doctor checks for protein in your urine when you visit him. If small quantities of a particular protein, albumin, are found in the urine, it is referred to as microalbuminuria. Your doctor may then recommend a drug known to reduce the risks of further kidney damage. A few people with advanced kidney damage may need dialysis (artificial kidney) treatment, or even a kidney transplant. Once again, prevention is the key. The lower the blood (or urine) glucose and the lower the blood pressure, the better the chances of avoiding this problem.

Infection

Infection, particularly of the skin and urinary system, is more likely to occur in people with diabetes than in people without diabetes. In addition, healing of even minor injuries is sometimes slower. These problems are more likely to occur if your diabetes is not well controlled. Once infection occurs, it is essential that your diabetes control is improved to assist in the healing process.

Foot ulcers

Foot ulcers are a particular risk. If feeling is lost, it is all too easy to be unaware of pressure on a toe or a minor injury. Repeated damage to this area, particularly if your blood circulation is poor, can then result in an ulcer. This can become more infected, producing swelling, redness and pain, and loss of control of your diabetes. You could become seriously ill, and even gangrene may develop, requiring amputation of part of your foot. Chronic ulcer infection can also damage the underlying bone, causing osteomyelitis. Once this sets in, long-term antibiotic treatment or surgery to your foot may prove necessary. Prevention is all-important; please read the answer to question 26 on pages 48–50 very carefully. If you develop even the smallest weeping blister, ulcer or sore on the foot, let your doctor or diabetes nurse know immediately.

All the above complications can be effectively treated, particularly if detected early. It is for this reason that doctors will make a systematic examination of various parts of your body approximately once each year. You may need to remind them that this annual review is due.

24

How important is my blood pressure?

Firstly, high blood pressure (hypertension) occurs rather more often in people with diabetes: around one third of all people with diabetes will need treatment for it at some time. It is important to avoid hypertension because it causes heart attacks and strokes, and can also worsen retinopathy and nephropathy. It is generally accepted that a blood pressure above 160/90 is undesirable in people with diabetes, and for most people with diabetes, lower targets are preferred. The UKPDS study mentioned earlier showed that achieving a blood pressure of 140/80 reduces both heart attack and stroke risk by 50 per cent. At this level, the retinas and kidneys are protected as well. You must make sure that your doctor or nurse checks your blood pressure at least once each year. Quite simple tablet treatment is available for this problem. If you are taking such tablets, make sure that your blood pressure is checked every three months or so. You should know what your blood pressure is, and also know what level your doctor is aiming for (it is a good idea to keep records of your blood pressure as well as your blood or urine glucose levels). Your doctor may feel that it is a good idea for you to check your own blood pressure from time to time. The equipment needed is not expensive, is reasonably accurate and is also quite easy to use.

25

Do all people with diabetes get complications at some time?

No. There is good evidence that most of the above complications are much less likely to occur if the glucose, blood pressure and blood fat (lipid) levels are well controlled, and if weight gain is avoided. However, it must be admitted that with even the best control you may show one or other of the complications mentioned on pages 41–6.

26

How important is foot care?

If you have diabetes, your feet can be very vulnerable. Nerve damage (neuropathy) can prevent feeling an injury, scratch or cut; poor blood supply to the feet may then mean poor healing of the injury and infection, or gangrene can develop. It is important to observe the following rules:

* Avoid walking barefoot, even at home.

* Do not cut your toenails too short, and cut nails to follow the line of the toe.

RIGHT **WRONG**

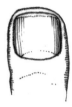 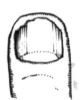

* Never cut your own toenails if you have a significant eyesight problem, or a nerve or blood vessel disorder affecting the feet. See a state-registered chiropodist regularly every six to eight weeks, if possible.

* Avoid tight shoes. Preferably have new shoes fitted by an expert who knows you are diabetic.

* Wash, dry and examine your feet carefully at least every other day: even the most minor infection should be immediately discussed with your doctor.

❖ Never attempt to treat any foot problem yourself; permanent damage may result from the use of over-the-counter remedies. Always seek professional advice first.

If an ulcer, sore or other foot infection develops, do not delay: contact your doctor immediately. Do not try to look after it yourself.

27

How will diabetes affect my lifestyle?

Can I smoke?
No. Diabetes alone may damage the blood vessels of your body, as mentioned earlier, causing strokes, heart attacks and exceptionally gangrene. If you smoke as well, your chances of such damage are very much greater.

Can I drive a car?
Yes, but the licensing authorities may want to have your doctor's reassurance that your diabetes is sufficiently stable and that you are otherwise well. An appropriate form will need to be completed, on which you must

mention that you have diabetes. On the whole, neither heavy goods (HGV) nor public service vehicles (PSV) can be driven by people with diabetes whose treatment puts them at risk of having hypos.

Can I play sport as usual?
Yes. See question 10 on page 23.

Can I drink alcohol?
Yes but, as mentioned earlier, calories do count. Excessive drinking can cause you to gain a lot of weight over time. Alcohol (especially spirits) may cause you to have low blood glucose levels (hypos), especially if you are not eating at the same time. Remember that you should always have a carbohydrate snack if you have an alcoholic drink.

Does diabetes interfere with employment?
Hardly. Jobs involving physical responsibility for other people (such as bus drivers, airline pilots and certain branches of the armed forces) are not appropriate if you are taking the sulphonylurea group of drugs or insulin (which are the only drugs that can produce hypos). The earlier discrimination against people with diabetes is now almost non-existent

since it has been shown that the work
record of people with diabetes is as
good as non-diabetics.

Can I get life insurance?
Yes. You may have to accept a 'loading',
but life assurance is possible for most
people with diabetes. Shop around and
seek the advice of your British Diabetic
Association office.

28

What about children?

Diabetes is at least partly inherited.
If either parent suffers from
diabetes, the risk of any one child
becoming diabetic at some time of
their life is certainly greater. It is worth
suggesting to your children that they be
regularly checked for diabetes once
they are above 40 years of age. It is also
sensible for them to make great efforts
to avoid becoming overweight, which
could trigger off their diabetes.

Pregnancy

If you are a woman in the child-bearing age group, you will be advised to be absolutely sure that your diabetes is perfectly controlled before becoming pregnant. Wait until your doctor gives you the go-ahead. Once you are pregnant, you will almost certainly need to have insulin injections for much of the pregnancy in order to achieve the level of control known to be important to ensure a healthy baby. Insulin can be discontinued again in most people after the confinement.

Pregnancy in a diabetic should always be managed by a physician/obstetrician team accustomed to dealing with diabetic pregnancies. A lot of emphasis will be placed on making sure that your diabetes is well controlled as this will reduce the risk of pregnancy complications.

Contraception

Most of the presently available low-dose pills are satisfactory for people with diabetes and there is no reason why you cannot use an intra-uterine device (IUD) or other contraceptive methods. If you are taking the contraceptive pill, it is useful to stop it and to have one normal period before you conceive, so that the exact duration of your pregnancy is known. Your doctor or diabetes nurse will be happy to discuss any other aspects of diabetes and pregnancy with you.

29

Are any other members of my family likely to get diabetes?

Yes. The risk of brothers and sisters being diabetic is about one in ten. A further one in five have a milder degree of blood glucose abnormality and may be more than usually prone to large blood vessel damage such as heart attacks. Your doctor may advise them to have a check-up.

When should I see my doctor or clinic nurse?

Routinely. Ideally you should have a discussion with a doctor or nurse at least every four months. Do not forget to take your test record book with you when you go.

At about yearly intervals and perhaps more frequently, your doctor will systematically examine your eyes, blood pressure, heart, blood vessels on the feet, and check for nerve damage. It is a good idea to remind your local surgery when your 12 months check is due. The doctor will test the urine for protein and check the level of control of your diabetes, your blood pressure and your kidney function. A blood sample is likely to be taken to see whether the blood fat (cholesterol and triglyceride) levels are normal. An alteration to your diet, and perhaps tablets, may be suggested if they are not.

In an emergency, if your tests show consistently high glucose levels, or if you begin to feel thirsty or unwell, do not wait – get advice. Make sure that you have one or more telephone numbers that you or your family or friends may contact for help and information on such unexpected problems, and write them down in the space provided on page 60. Your doctor may have given you another type of test strip (Ketostix) to measure ketones in the urine. Ketones will appear in the urine when fat is broken down to provide reserve energy. This may happen even in someone who does not have diabetes if they have not eaten for 12 hours or so. More important though, ketones appear in the urine of people with diabetes when control becomes really poor. Therefore, if you have consistently high glucose levels in urine or blood tests, it is a good idea to test for ketones. If the result is positive, contact your doctor or hotline (see page 59) immediately.

What should I do about identification?

Always carry a card or, better still, a bracelet or pendant, indicating that you have diabetes. In this day and age, accidents will happen, and it is obviously important that anyone can immediately identify you as having diabetes. The Medicalert Foundation (local address available from your doctor), which provides identification bracelets and pendants at a modest cost, now has branches in many countries. This system is highly recommended. Alternatively, have your local jeweller make up one for you.

Where can I get support?

Remember that finding out all about your diabetes is your responsibility. Your doctor, dietitian, diabetes nurse or chiropodist/podiatrist will be only too happy to answer queries and suggest further reading material.

Being a member of the British Diabetic Association has much to offer. It can help you follow recent trends in diabetes care. Much research into diabetes is also being carried out. You will find it useful and interesting to keep in touch with important developments that may relate to your needs.

Hotline number

Keep a record here of a telephone
number from which you can get
advice 24 hours a day, seven days a
week, should any sudden problem
occur which affects your diabetes. Your
doctor or diabetes nurse will advise
you which number to insert.

| |
| |

Other important contact numbers.

Your family doctor

. . . .

Your hospital clinic

. . . .

Your dietitian

. . . .

Your chiropodist/podiatrist

. . . .

Your diabetic advisory service

. . . .

Diabetes UK
020 7323 1531

Some books for further reading

Living with Diabetes – Type 2 by J. Day
(John Wiley and Sons)

Diabetes at Your Fingertips by P. Sonksen,
C. Fox and S. Judd
(Class Publishing)

Creative Recipes for All Occasions
(BDA Publications)

Real Food for Diabetics by Molly Perham
(W. Foulsham)

Index